SURVIVAL OF THE FITTEST

Written by Tommy Rozycki

Illustrated by Jennifer Slack

Table of Contents

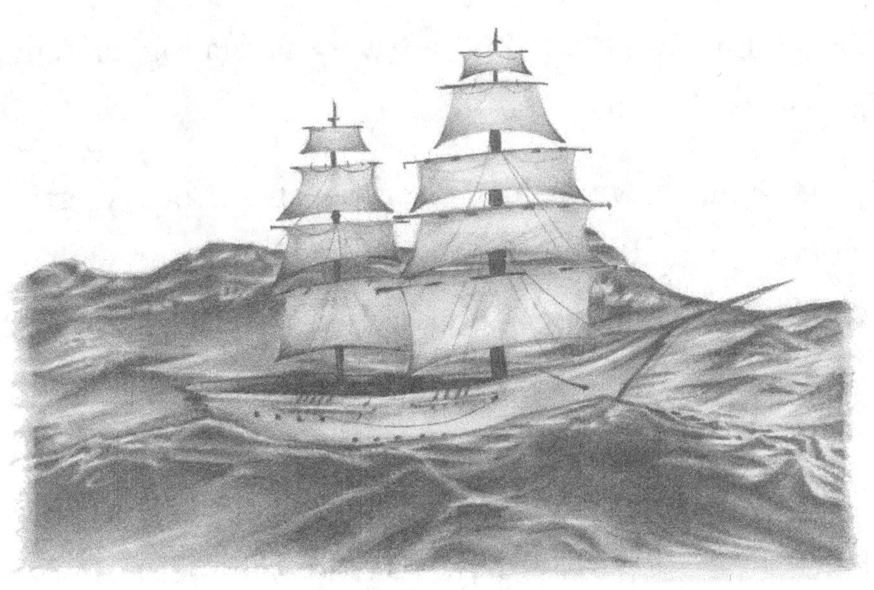

Chapter 1

Years ago, far out to sea, a small ship was making a rather large journey across open waters. Aboard this vessel, were a captain, his crew, and their passengers: a wealthy couple and their only son.

The family was heading from Cape Town, South Africa to Melbourne, Australia for a quiet vacation getaway. For days, the weather had been ideal for travel and the seas could not have been more agreeable. Spirits were high and all seemed well for the travelers. However, what the captain of the ship did not realize was that he was navigating directly into a terrible storm.

In what seemed like no time at all, heavy, gray clouds formed overhead and the sky became violent with roaring thunder and crashing lightning. Before they knew it, the crew and passengers were being tossed around as wave after giant wave slammed against the sides of their vessel. The ship creaked and cracked as the storm continued to pummel the boat for what seemed like hours.

The family huddled together on the deck of the ship as they witnessed men and supplies being forced overboard by the unrelenting barrage of wind and water.

The terrified, young boy looked around frantically at his surroundings trying to understand what was happening. But before he could make sense of it all, the last thing he saw as everything went black, was one final, giant wall of water heading their way.

There is no telling for how long the boy drifted or how far he traveled on that large piece of wood which had once belonged to the ship. His body must have realized it was no longer drifting among the waves, but had found itself washed up onto an empty beach.

As he began to open his eyes, the boy heard the sound of waves breaking on the shoreline and became aware of the warm sand he was now laying on. His head hurt, the bright sun bothered his eyes, and every muscle in his body seemed to ache. He attempted to stand to get a better look of where he was, but could only manage to make it to his knees.

The beach seemed to stretch on for as far as the boy could see. At the top of the white sand, a short distance away, was a massive jungle unlike anything he had ever seen! The boy rubbed his eyes unsure if this was real or if it was all a dream.

Once he felt some of his strength returning to him, the boy made his way towards the trees to relieve himself from the blazing heat of the sun. His skin was dry and he had never felt so thirsty in his entire life. He had learned from the captain of the ship that water from the ocean is not for drinking, so he knew that he had to find a stream or a lake if he was to quench his thirst.

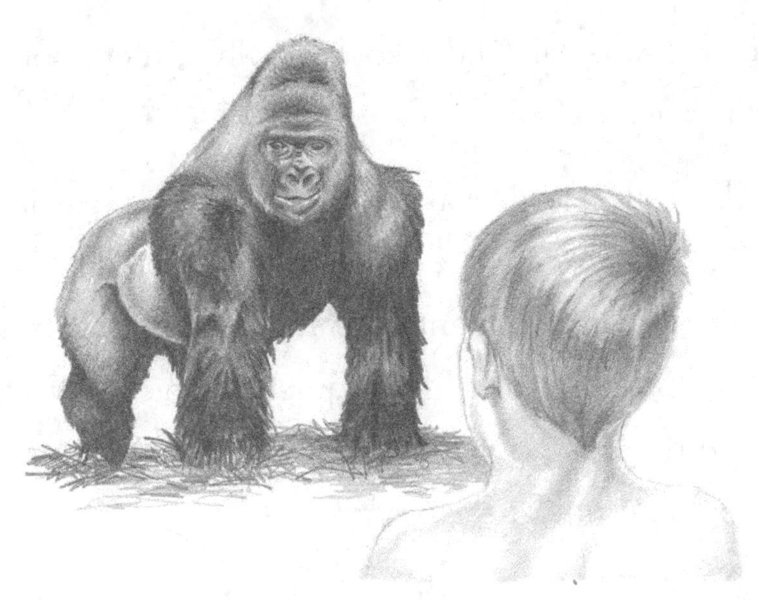

Chapter 2

As he made his way into the tropical forest, the boy pushed through all kinds of bushes as he stepped over sticks and stones with his bare feet. He was exhausted, but he knew he must continue to search for water before lying down to rest somewhere.

The shipwreck and his journey in the waves left the boy wearing nothing but his tattered, tan pants; his shirt and shoes had been lost somewhere along the way. The boy had short, light brown hair and fair skin. He was tall and also naturally athletic-looking for his age.

The boy hadn't traveled very far into the jungle when, suddenly, he heard something rustling in the bushes directly in front of him. Whatever it was, it was coming towards him quickly, and it was *big*. Before the boy could find a place to hide, a massive gorilla burst out of the woods!

Speechless and petrified, the boy was unable to run or yell for help. The giant ape stood over the boy calmly and looked at him curiously. What happened next shocked the boy more than anything else that had happened so far; the gorilla spoke!

"Hello, child. What are you doing here? Are you hurt?" asked the gorilla in a concerned, yet gentle voice. The boy, quivering in fear, was unable to respond. Again, the gorilla asked, "Are you hurt? What is your name?" With a shaken voice, the boy responded, "I-I, m-my name is D-Darwin."

"Hello, Darwin. Please, tell me, are you harmed in any way?" the ape asked yet again. As he began to calm himself, the boy answered, "No, I don't think so. I'm just very thirsty and I do not know where I am!"

"It is alright. My name is Gamba. Do not be afraid, child. Tell me what has happened and how you came to our island." In a confused state, Darwin exclaimed, "I-I'm on an island?"

Next, the young boy did his best to tell the gorilla all he could remember about his journey, his parents, and the storm.

"My, my boy, you *have* been through quite a bit of trouble. You *must* be exhausted. Let me take you somewhere for you to drink and then you may rest" explained Gamba.

The gorilla placed the child on his back gently and carried him off to a nearby stream. Upon arriving at the fresh water source, Darwin immediately hopped to the ground, ran to the water, and drank to his heart's content. The boy was so delighted and so busy quenching his thirst, that he did not realize he was being studied by someone just a few yards away.

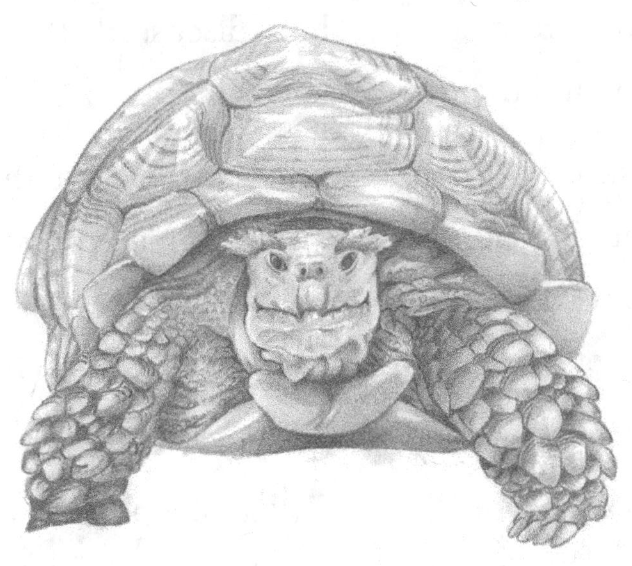

Chapter 3

Nearby, sitting atop a flat rock in the middle of the stream was a large tortoise. His broad shell was a magnificent sight and his bushy, gray eyebrows suggested to Darwin that he was rather old.

"Ahhh, Gamba, my dear friend, who is this young companion of yours? And how did he come to be here?" inquired the elderly tortoise, as he squinted his eyes to focus on the boy. Again, Darwin could not believe what he was seeing. The boy observed the two creatures as they discussed the strange situation and their unexpected visitor.

Eventually, Gamba turned to address the child, "Darwin, it is my pleasure to introduce you to Master Tafiti. His name means 'Knowledge Seeker', he is the island's oldest inhabitant and the wisest creature I have ever known."

"How do you do, sir?" Darwin politely asked as he bowed. Tafiti responded, "I do just fine, my boy. It is quite pleasing to still be surprised when you are as old as I am." Hesitantly, Darwin inquired, "How old *are* you exactly? If you don't mind me asking." The tortoise closed his eyes and took his time to answer. It seemed as if Tafiti was reflecting on all he had experienced and learned over his vast lifetime. After a brief pause, he opened his eyes and with a warm smile responded, "I am 135 years old. And I hope to see 150, as many tortoises do."

Dumbfounded by his answer, the young boy tried to think of what to ask the wise, old tortoise. But, before he could speak, Tafiti seemed to know what he was thinking already and said, "Yes, child. I have seen and done much during my time here, and now, I would like to help *you* if I may." "Oh, would you? That would be wonderful!" exclaimed Darwin.

"As you wish" replied Tafiti, "Now, do exactly as I say, and I will teach you an important lesson that will help you overcome your problems, no matter what obstacles you face in life." Tafiti nodded towards a smaller stone directly in front of him, also in the middle of the stream. "Join me, child" instructed the wise teacher.

Darwin gingerly tiptoed through the clear, cool water until he stood on the flat stone facing the large reptile. "Take a seat, close your eyes, and make yourself comfortable" the tortoise explained gently as he too closed his eyes.

Darwin obeyed and closed his eyes, awaiting further instruction. After a couple of minutes or so, Darwin impatiently opened one eye to see what was happening.

Tafiti was lying there with his eyes closed, appearing not to be doing anything. "Excuse me, sir. D-Did you fall asleep? What am I supposed to be doing?" Without moving or opening his eyes, the old master responded, "Keep your eyes closed, breathe slowly, and *clear* your mind. You have been through a great deal of trouble, my boy." After a short pause, a confused Darwin replied angrily, "How is sitting here with my eyes closed supposed to solve my problem? I need to find my parents! I need to get off this island! I need to get home!"

"Patience, my boy, you must have patience. Until you calm down and focus your mind, you will not accomplish anything worthwhile," explained Tafiti. "Your mind is a powerful tool and you must learn to use it properly. Focus on the problem at hand. How did you get here? Where do you need to go? And what must you do to get there?"

Darwin attempted to respond, "I nee-", but before he had a chance to answer, Tafiti interrupted "Do not speak. Think!"

With this command, Darwin attempted once again to follow his teacher's instructions. He did his best to remain calm with his eyes closed as he thought about the predicament he was in. Gradually, with each passing breath, Darwin felt more at peace, as his mind slowly became clear enough to think straight for the first time since he awoke on the beach. One by one, the events fell into place in his mind: the ship, his parents, the storm, and everything else that had led him to this moment.

After a short time, Darwin was brought back to the present moment by his teacher's voice, "Now, my child. Tell me what your mind has revealed to you." Darwin inhaled a calm, deep breath and replied, "Well, my parents and I were on a boat heading to Melbourne for vacation. We were coming from my home in Cape Town. Everything was going just fine until a terrible storm ruined everything. Oh, it was quite frightening! Before I knew it, I woke up here on the beach and then Gamba found me shortly after."

The tortoise took a moment before responding, "Hmmm. I see. Well, it so happens that I have both good news and bad news for you, young Darwin" said Tafiti. "This island is only a day or two's journey by sea to Melbourne. It is quite possible that your parents are already there looking for you." Darwin hopped up to his feet and exclaimed, "Am I really that close? Oh boy! Mom and Dad must be terribly worried about me."

"Calm yourself, my boy. Remember, losing control of your emotions will not help you solve your problems" explained Tafiti. "Although you are not far away from your destination, there is no way off of this island. You are just a boy after all."

Discouraged by the thought of being stuck on the island, Darwin stood up, turned around, and crossed the stream back to where Gamba was waiting for him. His head hung low and he had nothing to say.

"Young Darwin," said the old tortoise, "remember the lesson you have learned here today. Any time you are feeling lost or unsure, clear your mind and focus on the problem. You must *find* a way back to your parents. Farewell."

Darwin bowed to the wise master before Gamba placed him on his back once again. "Now, Darwin, I will take you somewhere safe for you to rest." Then, Gamba carried his new friend off into the jungle, as the young boy's eyes grew heavy and, eventually, closed as he drifted off to sleep.

Now it's *your* turn to practice Master Tafiti's lesson! Begin by sitting up tall, crossing your legs comfortably, and closing your eyes. Breathe in slowly and count to yourself for 5 seconds. Next, breathe out for 5 seconds and repeat. Do your best to relax, stay still, and "clear your mind." Try to practice this for 5-10 minutes every day!

Remember, Tafiti has had over *100 years* to practice this technique, so don't get discouraged if it takes you a while to get used to it!

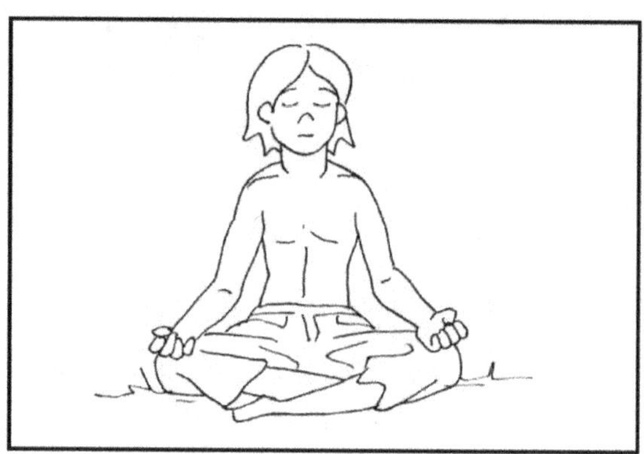

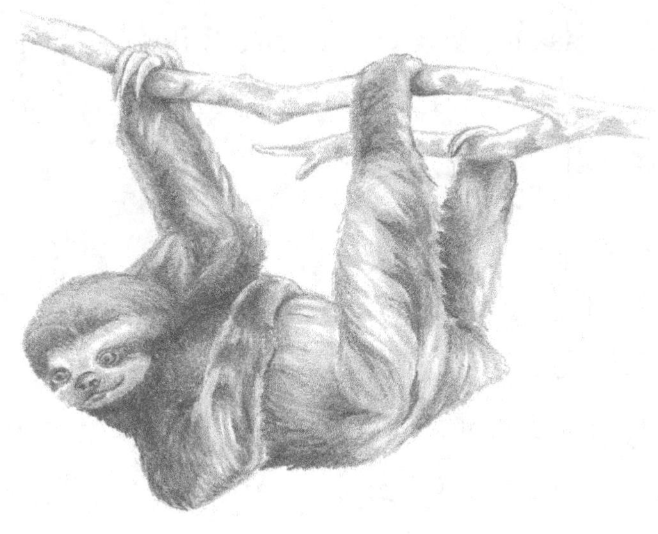

Chapter 4

When Gamba woke up later that evening, he heard a troubling sound off in the distance. Almost immediately, he realized it was Darwin, and it seemed as if he was struggling with something. They had lain down to rest together, so he was surprised when he awoke and did not see the child next to him. Although the ape was quite large, he rose to his feet quickly, and ran off to find the boy.

When he came to where he heard Darwin making all of the noise, Gamba couldn't believe what he saw. Darwin was adding vines to a pile he had already started and had pushed a couple of small tree logs next to each other.

"Darwin, what are you doing, boy? Haven't you slept at all?" questioned the gorilla. "I did for a short while Gamba, but I do not have time for sleep. I am building a raft. I must get back to my parents," replied Darwin. Gamba noticed the child was exhausted and must have been working for hours. "Darwin, it is important that you rest. You will not be able to go on like this for very long if you do not get some sleep."

"What's going on? ... Who is making all of that noise?" came a curious voice out of seemingly thin air. Darwin looked around, confused, because he did not see anyone and had not heard anyone approaching.

"Just a minute... I will be right down," said the strange voice. At this, Darwin looked up into the trees while Gamba simply smiled. "Who said that?'

asked Darwin. "You will see soon enough" chuckled Gamba.

After a few minutes of waiting, Darwin saw a small head covered in black and brown fur poke out from one of the treetops above them. In another minute's time, the entire body of a three-toed sloth revealed himself to the two friends.

"Hello, child… my name is Shu… What is it that you are doing down there?" asked the sloth. Darwin was unsure if it was because he was tired or not, but it seemed as if the slow-moving sloth took long, drawn out pauses in the middle of his sentences. The boy found this to be quite amusing but did not want to be rude and laugh at his new host.

"I am terribly sorry for disturbing you, but I am stranded on your island and I am desperately trying to get back to my parents," explained Darwin. "I figured, if I build a raft, I will be able to sail to Melbourne and meet them, but it is proving to be quite difficult."

Shu also noticed how tired the young boy was and could tell he was in need of rest. "Gamba… it has been a long time since I have seen you… I see you spend your time… with more interesting company these days… How long has it been… since this boy last slept?"

"Good evening, Shu. It is good to see you. I was just pleading with Darwin here to get a good night sleep before continuing with his plan. Maybe *you* can get through to him?" said Gamba.

"Ah, yes… Humans always seem… to be in a hurry. Work, work, work… Never any time to rest… If only they knew… how important it is… to rest," said Shu as he began to yawn.

Darwin replied, "Really? What's so important about sleep? Mom always wants me to get to bed at the same time every night, even when I don't feel like it!"

"Your mother sounds… like a smart woman, child… You should listen to her more often… You see… I may sleep anywhere… from 15 to 20 hours each day… but a child of your age… should be sleeping… about 9 to 11 hours a day…" explained the sleepy sloth.

Shu continued, "Proper sleep… strengthens the body… and sharpens the mind. It will help you grow… and give you plenty of energy… throughout your day… Do you understand, Darwin?"

"Yes, sir. I understand. But, shouldn't I work on my raft more? I must get off this island!" exclaimed the boy.

"In life… we do not rush… the things that matter the most to us. You must… Sleep well… Eat well… and Work hard… Follow these rules… and you will… return to your parents… in no time" explained the three-toed mammal.

Darwin thought about what Shu had said. The boy turned to his ape companion and agreed he should sleep before he continued to work on his raft.

"Thank you for your he-" but before Darwin could finish his sentence, he noticed the sleepy sloth had dozed off again right where he had been speaking only a few moments ago.

At this, Darwin and Gamba burst out in laughter together as they went to find a place to sleep for the night.

22

Now, let's see how *your* bedtime routine compares to what Shu taught Darwin!

At what time do you usually go to sleep at night?

What time do you usually wake up in the morning?

How many hours do you usually sleep?

How does this compare to the amount of sleep (9-11 hours) Shu told Darwin human children should sleep each night?

Do you have a bedtime routine that you complete every night? If so, what is it?

Shu's Tips for a Better Night's Sleep:

— Try to go to bed at the same time each night

— Keep your room dark and at a comfortable temperature

— Turn off your electronics 30 minutes before bed

— Practice deep breaths and meditating as you fall asleep

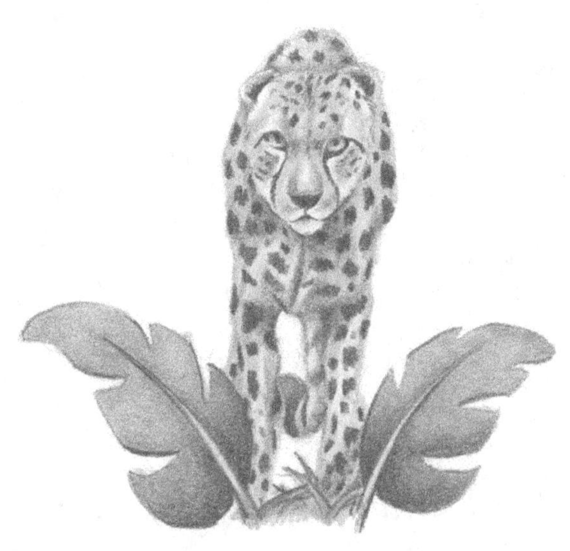

Chapter 5

The next morning, Darwin rose from his sleeping area feeling fully rested and alert. The first thing he did after he woke up was practice his meditation like Master Tafiti had instructed him to do.

After his meditation, the boy went straight to work on his raft. Sleep, meditation, work; this became Darwin's daily routine for quite some time. It was exhausting at times, but with the lessons he had learned from the tortoise and the sloth, Darwin was able to stay focused.

Darwin's top priority was returning to his parents. He missed them more and more with each passing day. Oh, what he wouldn't give to be held in the comfort of his mother's arms or to talk with his father in his study as they did almost every day at home. The boy refused to give up hope; he *must* return to them!

Gamba had been gone for days. He had explained to Darwin that there was someone he must go see on the other side of the island and that he would return to the boy as soon as possible.

Darwin's raft was coming along slowly. The hardest part of the process was finding and fetching the right logs. Once he had the wood, he would fasten the pieces together with vines that he found around the jungle. This was time-consuming, but the raft seemed like it would float once the time came.

One day, as Darwin was taking a short break to eat and drink some water, he heard a rustling in the bushes and two voices moving in his direction. The boy hid behind a tree because he did not want to leave his creation behind. Darwin slowly peeked around the tree to see who had found his raft. He knew running and abandoning all of his hard work was not an option. Carefully, he worked his way around the base of the tree and what he saw made his heart jump with joy!

It was Gamba! He had returned. And with him, stood a beautiful cat; unlike any animal Darwin had seen on the island. This majestic creature had a long, thick tail, big paws, and its tan fur was speckled with black spots.

"Darwin, there you are!" shouted Gamba "See, this is the boy I have been telling you about." Gamba said to the impressive feline.

"Gamba! Oh, how I've missed you!" replied the young boy. The gorilla said, "This is the friend I went to find. This is Chanah, she is a cheetah from the south side of the island." Simultaneously, the boy and the cat bowed to each other as a greeting.

Darwin pushed his unkempt hair out of his face as he welcomed the new guest to the northern part of the island. "It is so nice to meet you, Chanah!" shouted the boy. "The pleasure is all mine, Darwin," responded the graceful feline.

"The reason I left you and the reason I went to retrieve Chanah was because I decided you could use her help" explained Gamba. "Help with what?" asked Darwin. During their introductions, the boy hadn't noticed the feline had been studying everything about him. Within minutes, Chanah could see why the gorilla had come for her assistance.

Whether he was aware of it or not, Chanah noticed Darwin's body was worn down from day after day of hard labor. He was slightly out of breath and he was showing signs of fatigue.

Gamba turned to the cheetah, "Chanah, I believe you can explain better than I can." Chanah nodded as she stepped forward and said, "My child, you are exhausted from all of the hard work you have been doing. You must allow me to help you."

Darwin had to admit, even with the lessons he had learned from Tafiti and Shu, his work *was* catching up with him. Each day seemed a little harder to get through than the day before.

"But, how can you help me?" asked Darwin. In a nurturing tone, the female cheetah replied, "I would like to teach you to take better care of your body. You see, if you add exercise to your daily routine, your body and mind will grow stronger each day."

"But, shouldn't I save my energy for building my raft?" asked Darwin. Chanah replied, "Work and exercise are *both* important, so you must make time for both."

The feline continued, "I promise, if you exercise regularly, you will find your work to be much easier and you will also be more prepared for your journey back to your parents."

Darwin looked from Chanah to Gamba and he nodded his head showing that he understood what he must do. The next morning, Chanah taught Darwin a series of exercises that he could do every day to improve his stamina and help him stay alert throughout the day.

The cheetah stayed with the two friends for the next week to make sure the boy kept up with his routine. In what seemed like no time at all, Darwin noticed he had more energy each day and working on his raft was not as difficult for him anymore.

Eventually, Chanah had to return to her family on the south side of the island. Darwin thanked her for all of her help before she bowed, turned, and ran off swiftly into the bushes.

Regular exercise is not only important for Darwin, but for *you* as well! Can you complete a few of the exercises Chanah taught to Darwin?

Do your best to complete 10 reps of each exercise!

Inch Worms 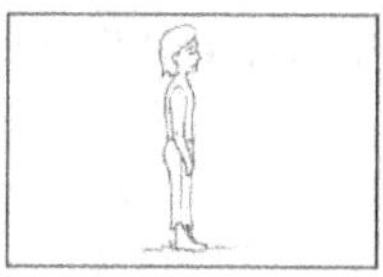 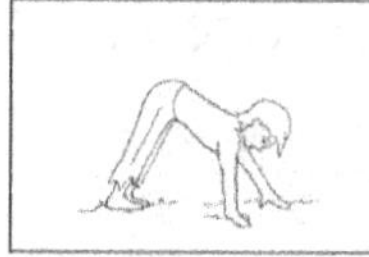 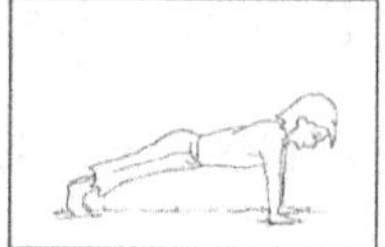

Mountain Climbers 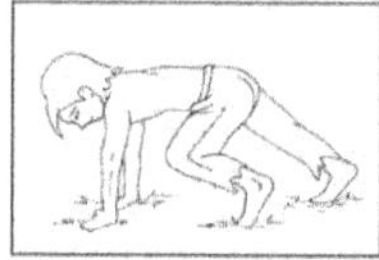 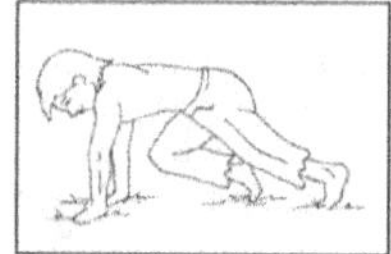

Jumping Jacks 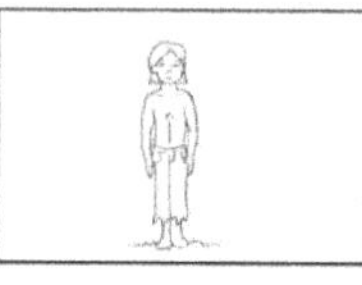 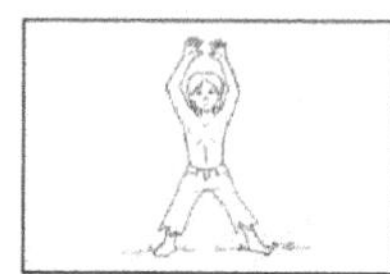

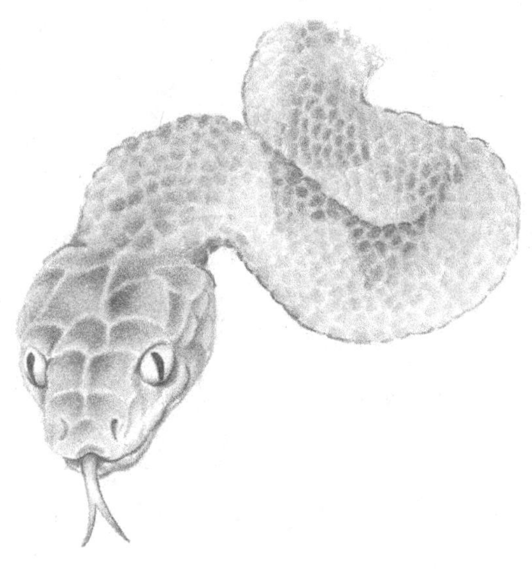

Chapter 6

One particularly hot day, after Gamba had returned from collecting food, he heard Darwin grunting and complaining about something over in his work area. The ape placed the food down and went to see what was troubling the boy.

"Darwin, is everything alright?" asked Gamba as he pushed through the bushes. Darwin placed a log down and replied to his friend, "I don't know what's the matter with me, Gamba. My body has been rather sore the past few days." The gorilla asked,

"Why haven't you mentioned anything to me?" Darwin responded, "I figured it would go away, but it hasn't. I feel a tightness, mostly in my neck, back, and legs."

Gamba took a minute to think to himself about what to do for his young friend. Darwin studied the gorilla's face and it looked as if he was having trouble making his mind up about something. "What is it, Gamba?" asked the boy.

Gamba explained, "There *is* someone who can help you. I can take you to her. Her name is Saabira and she lives in the center of the island. Many animals dare not to journey inland *because* of Saabira and her friends. She is neither friendly or trustworthy." After observing Darwin for a while longer and seeing how much the boy was struggling, Gamba decided they had no other choice.

"Saabira!" yelled Gamba, "I know you're here. Show yourself!" The two companions had found themselves in a dark part of the island, deep inside the jungle. The trees grew together so thick here, that the sun's light was barely able to reach the forest floor. Gamba had instructed the boy to stay very close to him around this part of the island. "You must act confident and do your best to show no fear," instructed the gorilla.

They both stopped walking as they heard what sounded like a whisper and a haunting laugh come from up above. Without thinking, Darwin jumped back and clutched Gamba's arm as he watched a giant snake circle and slither its way down a nearby tree. Her tough skin was yellow with a green diamond-like pattern along the back; she had piercing white eyes, and a red forked tongue.

Gamba gently removed the boy from his arm before cautiously approaching the snake to explain why they had entered her territory. When she spoke, Saabira dragged her S's in a most startling manner.

"S-S-So boy, in need of S-S-Saabira's help are you?" hissed the slippery serpent. Darwin shuddered in fright but tried to appear brave as he responded, "Y-Yes, I am." "Then why don't you s-s-step a little closer child and let S-S-Saabira have a proper look at you?" the snake invited, as she licked her sharp fangs with her forked tongue.

"That's enough, Saabira! Stop toying with the boy and show him why we are here" demanded Gamba. With a frightening chuckle, Saabira replied, "S-S-So be it…"

Darwin watched closely, almost hypnotized, as the snake began to contort her body in all types of shapes and forms on the ground in front of him. She moved this way and that, bending and twisting in ways Darwin had never seen before.

During her demonstration, Saabira said to the boy, "When we s-s-stretch often, we avoid injuring ours-s-selves. It is important to be flexible to remain s-s-strong and healthy without getting hurt. Saabira continued, "Now that you have s-s-seen S-S-Saabira s-s-stretch, it is your turn…"

After attempting to follow the snake's instructions for some time, Darwin started to become frustrated, "I can't do this! It is too difficult."

Saabira replied, "Yes-s-s, it is difficult, but s-s-so are many important things in life. Be patient, child." Darwin knew that he had to continue practicing if he was going to improve his flexibility, but he did not want to stay near the sinister snake a second longer.

"T-Thank you for your help, Saabira" said Darwin. Gamba nodded to thank the snake before they turned to head back to their area of the island. Saabira gave one last, long hiss before slithering off to her nearby cave.

From that day on, Darwin continued to practice the stretches Saabira taught him every day. Eventually, his flexibility began to improve and his body felt much better than it had before. He was now ready to finish his raft!

Flexibility is important no matter how old you are. It helps us to improve our strength and also to prevent injuries. So, let's see if *you* can s-s-stretch like a snake! Try some of these stretches that Saabira taught Darwin.

Perform each stretch for 15-30 seconds each!

Cobra Pose

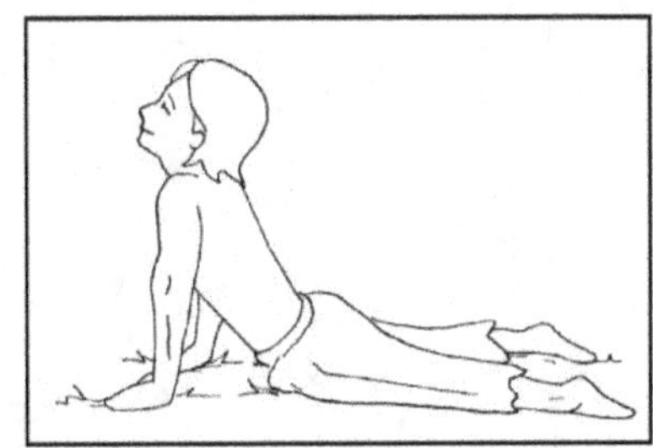

Butterfly Pose

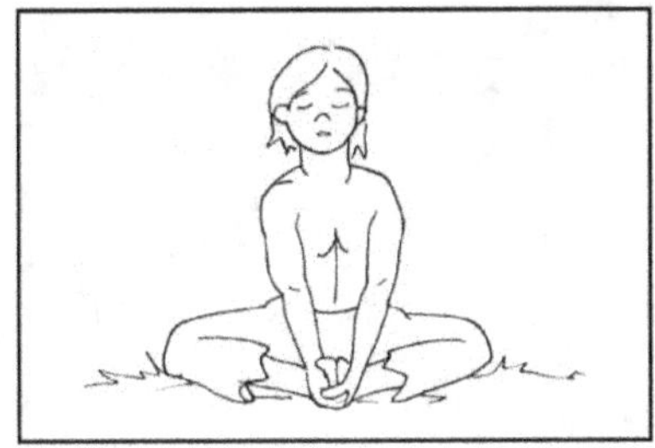

Child's Pose

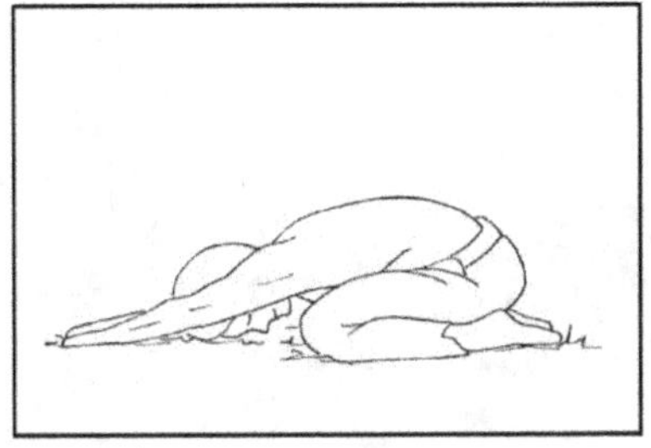

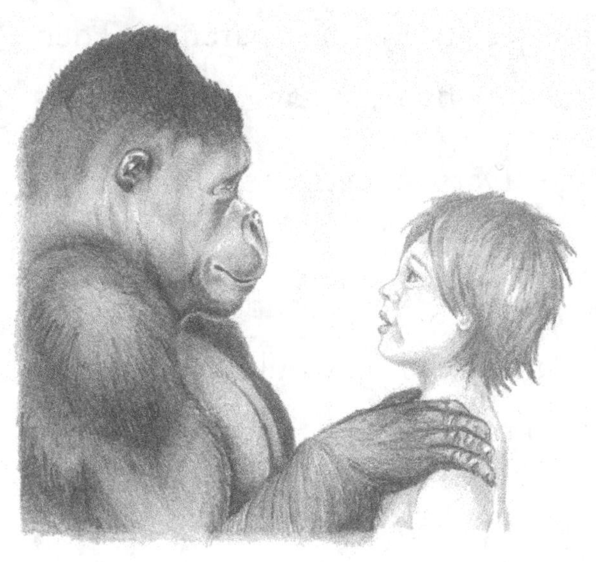

Chapter 7

Within a week's time, Darwin was putting the finishing touches on his raft. It consisted of eight wooden logs, which were fastened together by a number of sturdy, green vines. He had also carved an oar out of a small tree and built a sail with a red piece of canvas he had found washed up on the shore one day. Perhaps, from the same ship he had been on.

Darwin stepped back and marveled at his creation. He never knew he was capable of building anything like it. The raft seemed sturdy enough to withstand the journey back to his parents. Then, all of a sudden, the boy had a sinking feeling in his stomach.

You see, Darwin had been building his raft just inside the edge of the jungle in order to protect it from the sun, the wind, and the rain. But now, he realized just how far he would have to move the craft to get it into the sea.

The boy began to cry, "What have I done? I'll never be able to get this thing to the water!" He stomped his feet as he went to find Gamba.

"Oh Gamba! This is terrible. Just terrible!" exclaimed Darwin. "What is it, my boy?" asked Gamba curiously. The boy explained this new problem and asked if his friend would help him move the raft since he knew the gorilla was incredibly strong.

"I'm sorry, Darwin, but I will not help you," said Gamba matter-of-factly. Shocked at his answer, the boy's jaw dropped as he pleaded "But why not? Please, help me move the raft into the water!" The ape kindly explained, "This is something you must do on your own. You have come so far. Besides, you are stronger than you know." Darwin continued to plead, "B-But I have already tried to move it on my own and I can barely make it budge."

Gamba rose up from his seated position and approached the boy saying, "Allow me to teach you one final lesson, Darwin." The gorilla placed his large hands on the boy's shoulders and explained, "Strength, my dear friend, is not just about brute force, but also mental toughness as well." The boy stared at the gorilla confused as Gamba continued, "You have survived much and you have learned many lessons since your journey began. Consider all you have done while you have been on this island."

Darwin thought back on how much he had grown since he had washed up on the beach, feeling lost and frightened. He had learned, not only how to survive, but also the importance of taking care of his mind and body. Once the gorilla saw that the boy understood what he meant, they both nodded in agreement as Gamba said, "Now, about moving that raft…"

Without wasting any time, Gamba began teaching Darwin different exercises the boy would need to practice every day if he was to become strong enough to push the raft into the sea by himself.

Darwin was struggling with his workouts but he would not give up, Gamba believed in him. In the back of his mind, whenever he felt like giving up, Darwin thought of his parents' faces and this helped the boy push himself harder than ever!

The gorilla noticed great improvements in the boy's strength. Gamba was truly impressed with Darwin's determination.

In time, the boy could not believe how different he felt. He used Tafiti and Shu's lessons to stay focused and well-rested, while using Chanah, Saabira, and Gamba's lessons to make his body stronger. Darwin felt that the time had come; he was ready to leave the island.

Gamba taught Darwin many things during his time on the island, but showing him how to grow stronger may have been the most important lesson of all.

Can *you* complete a few of the strength exercises Gamba taught Darwin? Do your best to perform 10 reps of each exercise!

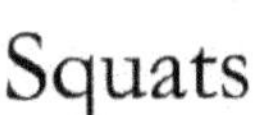
Squats
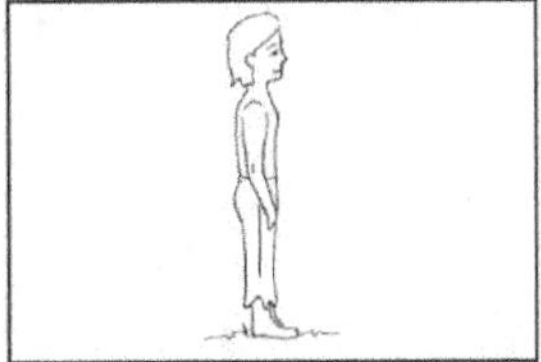
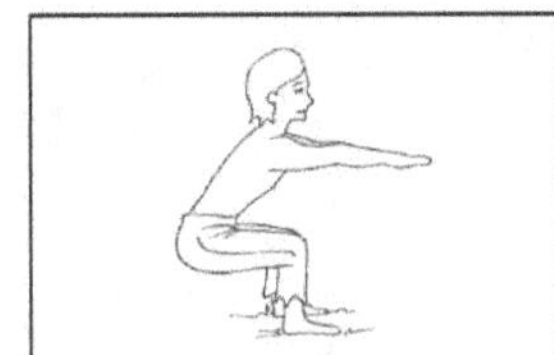

Lunges
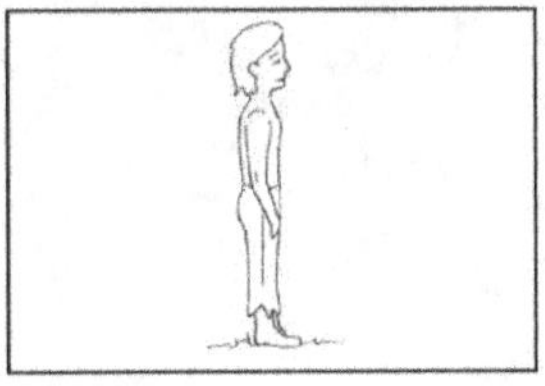
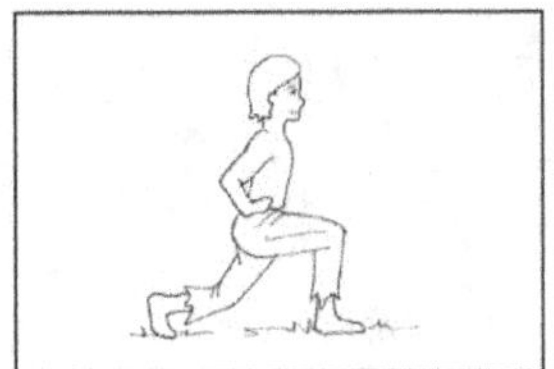

Push Ups
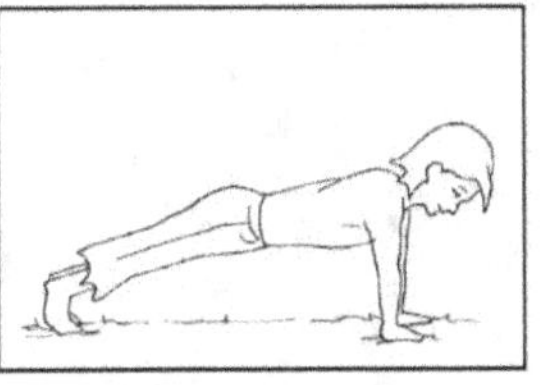
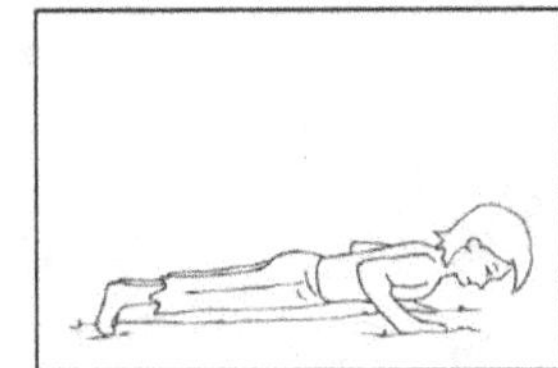

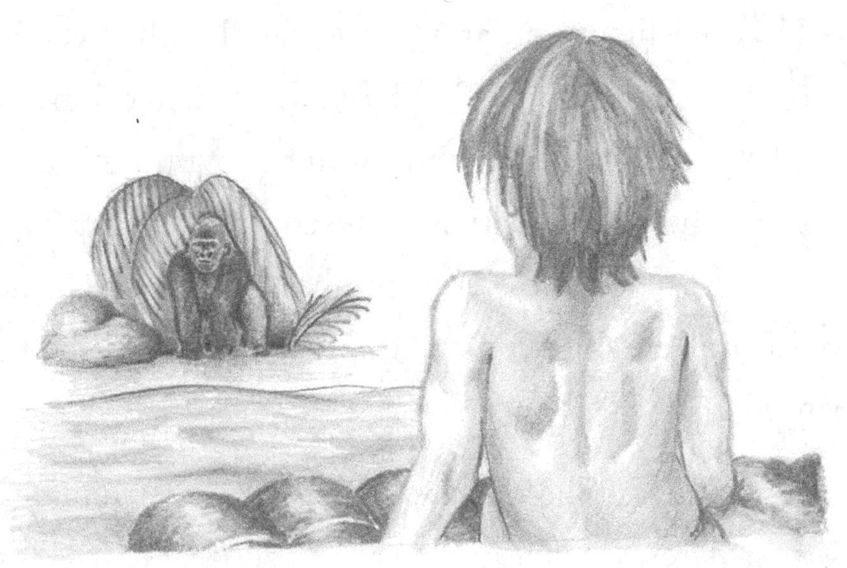

Chapter 8

The winds were strong that day and Darwin knew this would be to his advantage heading North towards Melbourne. All that remained now was to get his raft into the water, sail to the mainland, and find a way to reunite with his parents. After all he had been through, this final part of the journey did not seem too intimidating for Darwin.

With a deep breath, the boy placed both hands on the side of the raft and pushed with all of his might. To his surprise, the small vessel began to move!

He used his momentum and put all of his weight into each step, just as Gamba had instructed him to do. The gorilla stood by and watched with a pleased look on his face. Darwin refused to stop pushing until he reached the water because he was afraid he would not be able to get the raft moving again if he paused.

Once he felt the cool water rushing over his feet, Darwin knew he had reached the shoreline. At this moment, the boy knew what he must do next. Sadly, Darwin drew in a deep breath as he turned to say goodbye to the best friend he had ever known. Gamba had followed him every step of the way down the beach.

Darwin could not find the words to thank Gamba for all he had done for him. The gorilla placed one of his large fingers under the boy's chin and lifted it, "Do not be sad, Darwin. We both knew this day would come. You must return to the world and find your parents. I will never forget you." As soon as he said this, Darwin leapt into the gorilla's strong chest and cried, "I will never forget you either, Gamba!"

"You must go now, while the tide and the winds are in your favor," said Gamba. Darwin stepped back towards his raft slowly, knowing this would be the last time he ever saw his faithful companion. "Thank you, for everything" was the last thing the boy said as he hopped onto his raft and shoved off from the beach with his oar.

Darwin took one final look back at the island where he had learned so much about himself. He was grateful for all of the creatures he had met and for all of the lessons they had shared with him. But most of all, he was thankful for Gamba. He could still see the noble gorilla standing proudly on the beach as he sailed further and further away from the shore.

The boy shed a tear, because although he couldn't wait to be reunited with his parents, he would truly miss his new friend. And with that, Darwin turned towards the horizon with the wind at his back, ready to return home. He had survived, and he was stronger than ever.

The End

www.ingramcontent.com/pod-product-compliance
Lightning Source LLC
Chambersburg PA
CBHW051921250726
48659CB00002B/772